When
You
and Your Doctor
Pray

A Wellspring for Pregnancy,
Reproductive Health and Wellness

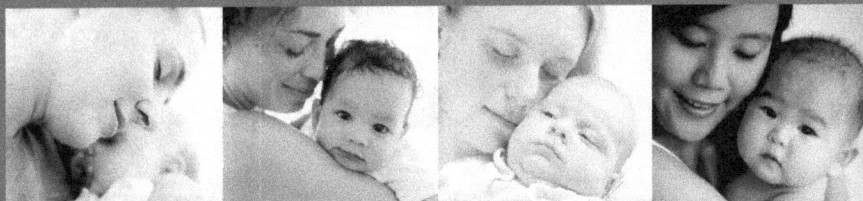

MIRONDA D. WILLIAMS, M.D.

When You and Your Doctor Pray

A Wellspring for Pregnancy, Reproductive Health and Wellness

MIRONDA D. WILLIAMS, M.D.

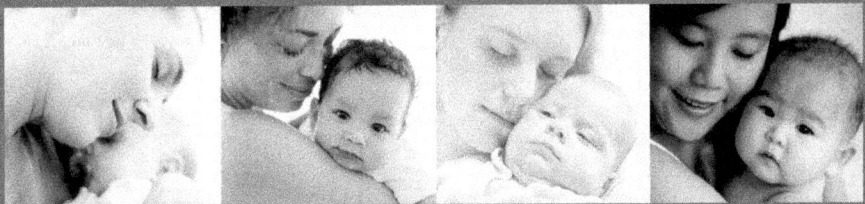

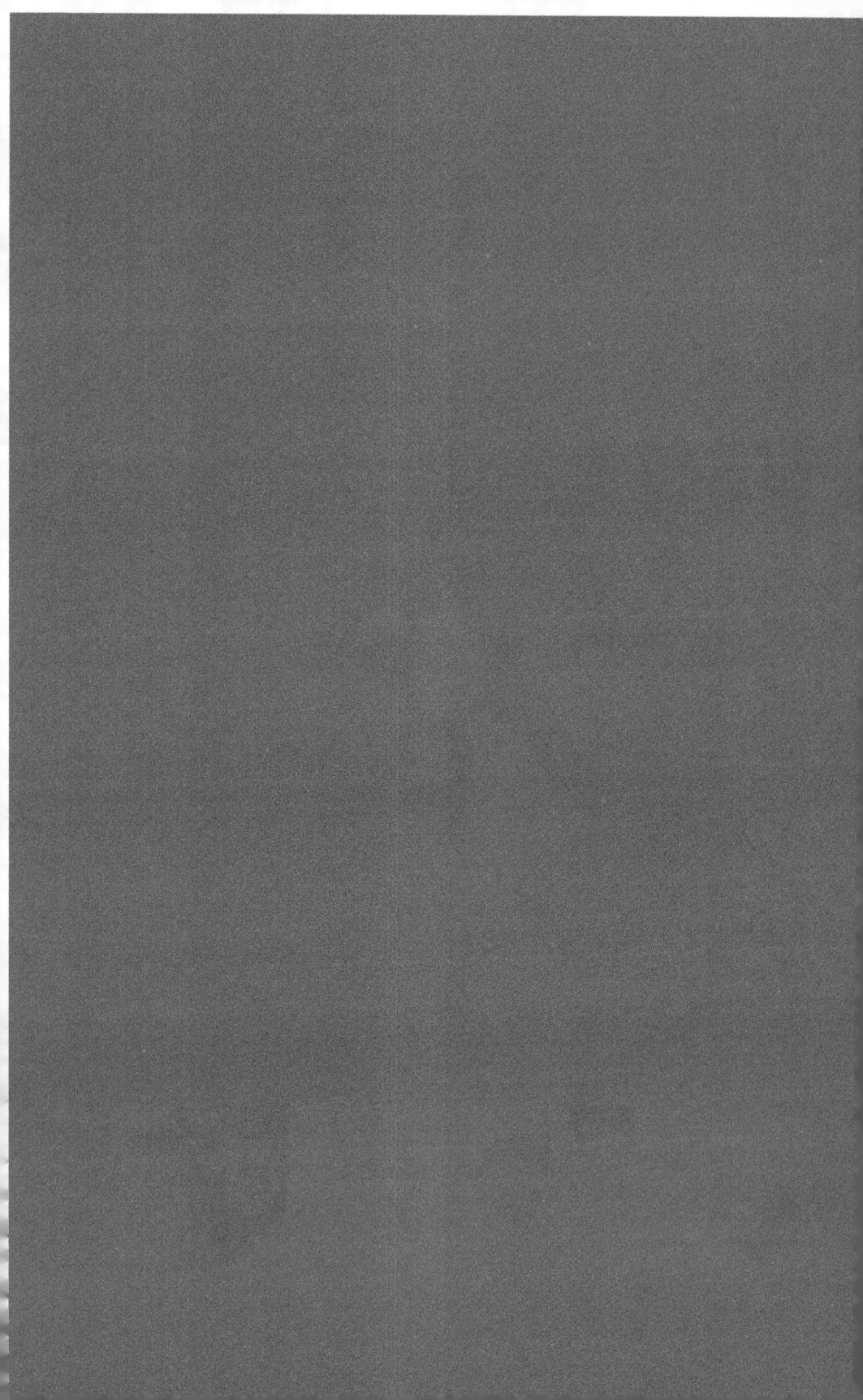

For my precious aunt Delores Freeland Yates,
who was a mother to many,
though she did not birth one.

For my marvelous grandmother Mattie Patterson Freeland,
who was a mother to an entire community.

And for my dear grandmother Ozie Green Williams,
who left us too soon but who lives on in her nine children
and numerous grandchildren and great-grandchildren.

May you all rest peacefully.

✂ *Acknowledgments* ✂

I first thank God for the privilege to write this work with His inspiration and guidance. I bless God for my parents Milton and Alice Williams, who introduced me to the power of prayer and inspired me to begin my prayer life. Many family members, friends and colleagues assisted with this work, most notably Leslie T. Fenwick, Ph.D. I am grateful for her insight and endless support throughout my writing process. Without her assistance, this book would not have been possible.

As with everything else in my life, I have not gotten to this point on my own. I acknowledge en masse all of my instructors, mentors and biblical teachers. Most importantly, I thank the Rev. Sharma D. Lewis, who helped to review early versions of this book. I am blessed to have been in her WISE (Women in Search of Excellence) Bible study at Ben Hill United Methodist Church in Atlanta for over eight years. I will always be indebted to her for imparting all that she has into my life.

There are also many women I have cared for over the years who have inspired me and taught me how to pray and believe God for miracles. I honor them all with this work. Three, however, deserve special mention: Angela Johnson, Rishal Dinkins-Stanciel and Felecia Freeman. These three women are the embodiment of what can happen when you and your doctor pray.

Angela Johnson taught me the real meaning of persistence and faith with her fight against the odds. She is now the mother of two beautiful boys after many early and tragic pregnancy losses. Her faith inspired my faith to greater heights. Through her journey, she showed me the real meaning of motherhood.

Rishal Dinkins-Stanciel was told that another pregnancy would be dangerous to her health because of the life-threatening complications that she had with her earlier pregnancies. However, God said, "Not so." She is now the mother of a third joyful blessing. Her story taught me how to believe in God's promises and to expect them to come to pass. She can also be credited for the idea for this devotional.

Felecia Freeman taught me to always praise God and believe, no matter what. Her giving birth against the odds is proof of God's abiding love and faithfulness.

Finally, I am deeply grateful to Tippi Hyde, The Editing Expert, for her conceptual and technical expertise, insights and enthusiasm for this project.

Scriptures in this book are taken from the Holy Bible. Bible versions are abbreviated as follows:

NIV—New International Version

KJV— King James Version

NKJV—New King James Version

❧ Contents ❧

❦ *Introduction* ❦

This collection of prayers evolved out of a mandate released in my spirit. That mandate was born out of traveling to Africa, which I believe to be my ancestral home. During my time there, the spirit of prayer and praise was awakened and ignited. I witnessed Africans walk for miles and wait for hours, even through the night, for the opportunity to untiringly praise God and to hear a rhema (fresh and timely word) from the Lord. That experience changed my life forever. I will never be the same.

I embarked on this endeavor with my earliest connection to prayer as a child at Wheat Street Baptist Church in Atlanta. Each Sunday would start with the congregation reverently singing,

"Sweet hour of prayer! sweet hour of prayer!

That calls me from a world of care,

And bids me at my Father's throne

Make all my wants and wishes known.

In seasons of distress and grief,

My soul has often found relief,

And oft escaped the tempter's snare,

By thy return, sweet hour of prayer!"[1]

Next, we would pray the Lord's Prayer. I offer this foundational prayer now for all caregivers and those who are entrusted in our care:

Our Father, which art in heaven, Hallowed be thy name. Thy kingdom come. Thy will be done in earth, as it is in heaven. Give us this day our daily bread. And forgive us our debts as we forgive our debtors. And lead us not into temptation, but deliver us from evil: For thine is the kingdom, and the power, and the glory, for ever. Amen.

Matthew 6:9-15 (KJV)

I believe that I have been given a special opportunity to speak very specifically to spiritual and physical conditions that affect women's health and reproductive capabilities. My obstetrical and gynecologic education has given me the

---

[1] *Sweet Hour of Prayer.* Lyrics by William Walford (1845). Music by William B. Bradbury (1861).

necessary tools to identify the physical manifestations of spiritual issues in women's reproductive health and well-being. My spiritual preparation has provided me with the knowledge and sensitivity to stand with women and their families to facilitate divine promises and to thwart the enemy. I am honored and humbled by what God has done with me and through me.

"... a spring of water welling up to eternal life."

John 4:14 (NIV)

God has given me a vision for medicine and miracles; I call it MD WELLSPRING. Using principles of sound medical science and spiritual disciplines can maximize the atmosphere for the miraculous to occur and for you to obtain your heart's desires. Your desires for health, healing and well-being may include optimizing weight management, fertility, gynecologic health and overall physical, emotional and mental health.

As Isaiah 58:11 (NIV) states, "The LORD will guide you always; He will satisfy your needs in a sun-scorched land and will strengthen your frame. You will be like a well-watered garden, like a spring whose waters never fail." God is the great physician, creator and designer of our bodies and of all of the intricate systems that work in concert to sustain life and health. Similar to the marriage covenant between God, husband and wife, a threefold cord is not easily broken. So it is in the relationship between a physician and the patient when both acknowledge God as the ultimate creator and sustainer of life.

The Bible states that some things come only through fasting and prayer. My approach to medicine is to work in those areas that need to be optimized physically as well as spiritually. God has shared His wisdom about maintaining our bodies and our health. He is truly our wellspring, that abundant source and resource from which we can continuously draw.

There are many areas where God's word can make an impact: diet, nutrition, physical fitness, emotional well-being, mental health, fasting, spiritual/Christian counseling and "dis-ease" identification. I use the term dis-ease to highlight the connection of disruptions in spiritual or emotional well-being to the physical manifestation of medical disorders, a disruption in the ease or balance of mind, body, spirit and soul by which we are divinely designed to function.

My experience has shown me that our concept of healing needs to address all aspects of our lives. My MD WELLSPRING vision for medicine and miracles is not just a prescription for patients to follow but one that the physician aspires to as well. The key intersection in this vision is passionate prayer that transforms individuals and circumstances.

Prayer involves the worship and adoration of God for who He is. Prayer acknowledges His character, majesty, sovereignty, mercy, goodness, grace and faithfulness. Prayer humbles us as we confess our sins and shortcomings and as we profess our submission to God's will and plan for our lives. In prayer we thank God for His mighty acts and salvation as well as lay our concerns before Him. Prayer is finding that secret place where we can quiet our spirits to hear God speak.

As our relationship with God grows and our knowledge and understanding of His word expands, we can declare His promises and decree His plans for our lives as the Holy Spirit reveals and guides. When all is said and done, our confidence is in knowing and accepting that God is God alone.

I know that I have been called by God to be a physician. Not only am I held to high professional standards as a physician, I am dedicated to using my education, talents and skills for those entrusted in my care, an awesome responsibility indeed. My higher calling in life is to pray with and for patients and the medical staff, administrators and other professionals in the medical facilities who partner in their care. God has gifted me medically to maneuver with my hands through skill and training, and just as importantly, He has gifted me spiritually to petition heaven for healing and wholeness through prayer.

Over the years I have witnessed God moving in the lives of many women who have struggled with pregnancy, labor and delivery, and I believe that I have a special sensitivity to these women. I have learned to never say "never," for with God all things are indeed possible. I know that God can provide for women today the same fulfilled promises He did for the biblical women Sarah, Hannah and Rachel many centuries ago.

The Bible is replete with scriptures that strongly encourage us to pray, both individually and corporately. Our communication with God draws us to Him. "Again, I tell you that if two of you on earth agree about anything you ask for, it will be done for you by my Father in heaven. For where two or three come together in my name, there am I with them" (Matthew 18:19-20, NIV).

There are many books of prayers and much scientific research about the physical and emotional impact of prayer and meditation on various medical conditions. There are also many books and manuals on the developmental stages of pregnancy that educate couples and prepare them for labor and delivery, as well as for the care of their newborn. However, I am not aware of any other works with prayers and medical insight specifically for reproductive health and pregnancy.

My heart has been touched to present this work at this time. My intention is to present a framework that marries the medical and spiritual components of wellness. The foundation of this framework is prayer, for the prayer of a righteous man or woman is powerful and effective (James 5:16).

Too many of us have been robbed of our health and destiny. Unfortunately, some of us have made destructive choices that aided in these poor outcomes. We can take back what has been stolen and make wise decisions as we move forward, toward our blessings. We can stand on the assurance given in the word of God referencing two or more agreeing in prayer. A special and powerful synergy exists when you and your doctor pray!

Part I: Prayers for Women at the Well

. . . and Jesus, tired as he was from the journey, sat down by the well. It was about the sixth hour. When a Samaritan woman came to draw water . . .

John 4:6-7 (NIV)

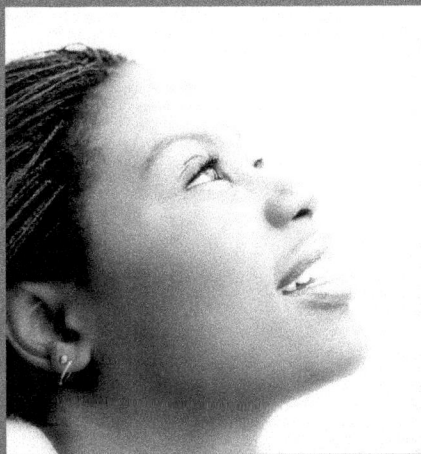
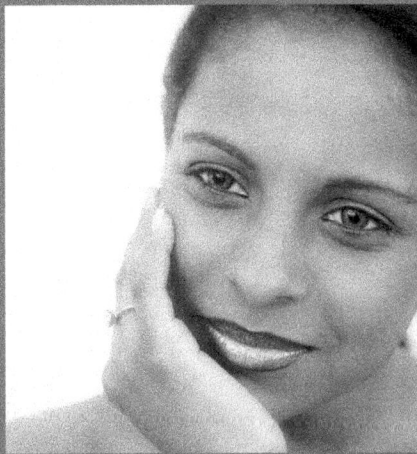

Jesus answered, "Everyone who drinks of this water will be thirsty again, but whoever drinks the water I give him will never thirst. Indeed, the water I give him will become in him a spring of water welling up to eternal life."

John 4:13-14 (NIV)

How glad I am that Jesus will still meet us at our point of need. It does not matter the circumstances that have led us to our present situation, Jesus is already waiting on us whenever we are in need, as He was for the woman at the well. Sometimes when we have filled a valid need (spiritually, emotionally or physically) from a seemingly obvious source, we find that there is still a void that only God can truly fill.

As a physician, I am acutely aware of the choices we make that negatively impact our general health and well-being and prevent us from enjoying all that God would have for us. These choices are generally related to nutrition, exercise and lifestyle. Though God is willing and able to step in, we must be willing to do what we know to be right and good for ourselves.

Many women have a myriad of responsibilities including social/civic activities, work, home, church and family. We do not do ourselves or those who depend on us any good when we neglect our health and well-being. The challenge we have is to achieve balance in the important areas of our lives.

Because of the nature of the practice, women share many intimate details of their lives with their obstetricians and gynecologists (OB/GYNs). Patients have cried in my office, and sometimes I have cried with them. They have expressed joy as well as hurt, fear and confusion about their busy lives, physical ills and emotional concerns.

My patients represent a wide spectrum of women: teen mothers; soccer moms; single parents; expectant moms who have had abortions in the past; women who were victims of physical or sexual abuse; promiscuous single women, some with histories of sexually transmitted diseases; and busy professional women juggling the demands of career and home.

With their varied lives, many of these women have complex histories that include regrets and bad habits and are in need of changing these habits and of physical healing. Many of them also deal with physical health concerns that center around their reproductive system: the uterus (womb), fallopian tubes, ovaries, hormones, muscles and the bone structure of the pelvic cavity. Often our physical healing process begins in the mind and spirit with forgiveness, for ourselves as well as for others.

"Come to me, all you who are weary and burdened, and I will give you rest. Take my yoke upon you and learn from me, for I am gentle and humble in heart, and you will find rest for your souls. For my yoke is easy and my burden is light."

Matthew 11:28-30 (NIV)

And without faith it is impossible to please God, because anyone who comes to him must believe that he exists and that he rewards those who earnestly seek him.

Hebrews 11:6 (NIV)

Part I:
Prayers for Women
at the Well

A Prayer for Forgiveness

Therefore, if anyone is in Christ, he is a new creation; the old has gone, the new has come!

2 Corinthians 5:17 (NIV)

O God, I bless You and will forever sing Your praise! I will lift Your name above all others. You are Yeshua, the Messiah, my savior. You went to the cross and died for my sins, then rose again to sit at the right hand of the Father. Therefore, I have been made new; old things have passed away.

You are my Kinsman Redeemer. You paid the ultimate price—just for me! I am able to forgive others for injuring me in the past. I am also able to forgive myself for my own choices that were outside of Your will for my life. I am able to move forward to the blessings You have for me.

You, blessed Savior, are Jehovah-M'Kaddesh (the Lord who sanctifies), who set me apart for sacred use. You purify. You edify. You love so that I can love myself completely and without reservation.

Your grace and Your mercy are overwhelming and all encompassing of past, present and future times.

Thank You for Your saving grace.

Thank You for Your keeping grace.

Thank You for Your purifying grace.

Thank You for forgiving me as I forgive all.

In You I am free!

Amen

℞

Meditate on release

Read Romans 8:1

Pray for understanding and discernment

A Prayer for Wholeness

And you have been given fullness in Christ, who is the head over every power and authority.

Colossians 2:10 (NIV)

O Thou Great Jehovah! You are Jehovah-Jireh (the Lord who provides).

You are El Shaddai (God Almighty).

There is none like You! I praise You and lift You above all things and situations. Your word says that You have come to give life and life more abundantly, above all that we could ask, think or imagine.

You designed my heart, mind and body to work in harmony. You designed my surroundings that I may do Your will and show Your glory. I must do all that You have called me to do. I cannot be hindered by anything—neither physically, emotionally nor spiritually.

Father, continue to speak life and correction where needed. Reveal Yourself to me. I am declaring that I will do what You have instructed me to do with my vocation, family, nutrition, exercise, recreation and rest. With You, God, I am well, whole and complete, lacking nothing in any area of my life! Though You have blessed me with knowledge, talent, ability and access to resources, I recognize that Your power alone is sufficient to save and heal.

I align my mind to Your mind that I may execute what You have shown me to achieve the wholeness and balance in my life that You desire. I cast down any apathy, excuse, confusion or chaos that may come to disrupt Your glorious plans for me to have a healthy mind and body.

I am fearfully and wonderfully made. I am positioned to receive wise spiritual counsel, appropriate medical consultation and the wisdom needed to manage busy schedules and numerous responsibilities.

As I stand with my healthcare providers, bless our homes, families, work environments and churches. Continue to bring us into our divine destiny as vessels of sacred service!

In Jesus' name.

Amen

R_x

Meditate on being fearfully and wonderfully made

Read Psalm 139:14

Pray for the capacity to be blessed

A Prayer for Lifelong Health

Dear friend, I pray that you may enjoy good health and that all may go well with you, even as your soul is getting along well.

3 John 1:2 (NIV)

O Lord, my God, You are my health and my strength.

No good thing will You withhold from those who walk upright before You (Psalm 84:11).

Grant me wisdom with which to frame my life. Give me clear direction so that I can be in pursuit of those things that I need to achieve my destiny. Keep me from activity that brings destruction to my body and soul.

Guide me in Your Word so that I will be able to stand on Your promises regarding good health, wholeness and well-being. You sent Your Word that has power to heal, and I know that there is still healing in Your wings and restoration in Your promises.

I stand with my healthcare providers to decree that I will not die. I will live, and I will declare the glory of the Lord. My doctor affirms that "God is within her, she will not fall. God will help her at the break of day" (Psalm 46:5, NIV).

I am so blessed to call You Lord, for You are faithful.

With You is the fountain of life, and through You, my days will be many and years will be added (Psalm 36:9).

Your glory, God, forever.

Amen

℞

Meditate on goodness and mercy all the days of your life

Read Psalm 23:6

Pray to finish strong and well

A Prayer for Sanctuary

"Fruit trees of all kinds will grow on both banks of the river. Their leaves will not wither, nor will their fruit fail. Every month they will bear, because the water from the sanctuary flows to them. Their fruit will serve for food and their leaves for healing."

Ezekiel 47:12 (NIV)

My Sovereign Lord, let the words of my mouth and the meditation of my heart be acceptable in Your sight (Psalm 19:14).

Allow the places of healing where I walk to flow with water from Your holy temple.

Let the gospel of Christ be preached through my life and behavior.

May I be a tree whose roots sink deep into Your good soil that I may bear all that You would have me to bear for Your divine will and purpose.

May I live long, prosper and be in good health as my soul basks in You.

Your glory is my destiny!

Amen

R_x

Meditate on being in a place of abundance

Read Psalm 66:12

Pray knowing God will supply

Part II:
Prayers for Gynecologic Health

Heal me, O LORD, and I will be healed; save me and I will be saved, for you are the one I praise.

Jeremiah 17:14 (NIV)

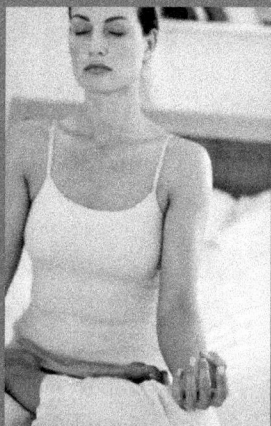

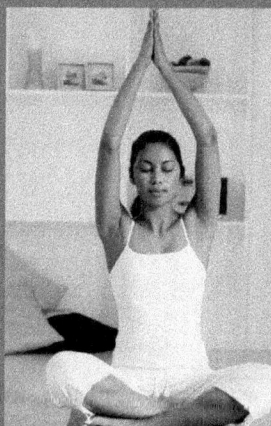

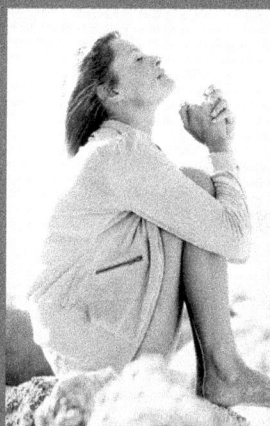

During my years of medical practice, I have seen stress and emotional issues manifest in symptoms of disease and pain in the pelvic area. Women can develop several abnormalities in various areas of their reproductive system including bleeding, pain and abnormal growths.

As gynecologists, it is our mandate to walk with women through their many phases of life, and we frequently have to manage various disorders over many years. It is our hope and prayer that every woman's life is filled with health and wellness. However, it is occasionally necessary to combat the ravages of unwise choices, time, physical injury or other external forces. We can give praise even in the most challenging circumstances ("yet praise") because ultimately our hope is in God, our savior (Psalm 42:11).

While writing this book, I was lead to many scriptures in the Bible that address healing and health. Jesus' ministry of healing on earth frequently involved the miraculous. Experience has shown me time and time again God's willingness and ability to supernaturally intervene in our physical circumstances. I am blessed to participate in God's healing process with the use of many medical and surgical techniques as well as with prayer.

Good medical care in the diagnosis and treatment of illnesses is essential. However, it is equally important to know that we have a source that goes beyond nature and medicine. We must use all of the resources at our disposal to prevent the evildoer from wreaking havoc in our lives. Thankfully we have God's word to use in our arsenal along with specific medical information about what may be affecting us physically or emotionally. God continues to miraculously heal and deliver just as He did when Jesus walked the earth and laid hands on the sick, opened blinded eyes and stopped the abnormal flow of blood.

. . . He welcomed them and spoke to them about the kingdom of God, and healed those who needed healing.

Luke 9:11 (NIV)

Part II:
Prayers for Gynecologic Health

A Prayer for Well-Being

When Jesus saw her, he called her forward and said to her, "Woman, you are set free from your infirmity."

Luke 13:12 (NIV)

O God, You are omnipotent, omnipresent and omniscient.

You are a sovereign God whose power is not diminished and whose hand still stretches forth to heal and deliver.

There may be one or more conditions that threaten my gynecologic health and provide challenges for all those charged with my care. Some of these conditions may be demonic attacks via generational, genetic or physical avenues and some, admittedly, because of my previous choices.

Your word says that You will restore the years to me and make my latter times greater than the former. You will provide strength to my body and health to my marrow (Haggai 2:9).

Speak through Your Holy Spirit, and give divine revelation and instruction to my doctors and me. Give me the discipline to do what You declare for the sake of my health and wellness, and give me wisdom to make the right choices.

I cast down any strongholds and devious plans or distractions.

By Your power, I break generational curses sent to decrease my quality of life.

By Your blood, destroy the weapons of cardiovascular, pulmonary, hormonal or central nervous system disruptions sent to compromise my body.

The weapons formed will not prosper (Isaiah 54:17)!

Breathe in me again, as You did in the beginning, the breath of life.

By Your stripes, I am already healed (Isaiah 53:5).

Move through my doctors' sound medical judgment.

Move by Your restorative miracles, corrective miracles and creative miracles!

In Jesus' name.

Amen

R~x~

Meditate on healing

Read Isaiah 58:8

Pray until something happens

A Prayer for Pelvic Pain

A cheerful heart is good medicine . . .

Proverbs 17:22 (NIV)

Dear God, give my healthcare providers divine insight and help them to show compassion as I work through this process of finding the problem and addressing the cure.

Infuse all medications and therapies with Your Holy Spirit.

Send Your healing balm to soothe and correct.

Do not allow me to become so consumed with the problem of pain that it becomes a stronghold that cripples and clouds my mind and emotions.

I align my mind and heart to Your mind and heart so that I will be able to see as You see and to speak my healing using Your word.

May Christ fill my heart, for out of the abundance of the heart the mouth speaks (Matthew 12:34)!

I loose (cast down) vain imaginings that exalt themselves above You to come against Your blessings.

In You I live!

Amen

R_x

Meditate on relief and comfort

Read 1 Chronicles 4:10

Pray for God's healing balm

A Prayer for Abnormal Bleeding

And a woman was there who had been subject to bleeding for twelve years, but no one could heal her. She came up behind him and touched the edge of his cloak, and immediately her bleeding stopped.

Luke 8:43-44 (NIV)

Then he said to her, "Daughter, your faith has healed you. Go in peace."

Luke 8:48 (NIV)

Dear God who sustains in the waiting periods and God of the sudden miracles, You are no respecter of persons. What You have done for one, You will do for another!

The menstrual cycle is a very precise coordination of a woman's anatomy, which is complex in form and function on its own. Therefore, there may be many abnormalities or areas open to attack that can disrupt Your divine design. No matter the complexity or duration of the problem, when I press my way to You, I will be healed.

The faith that heals is faith in Jesus alone.

Jehovah-Rophe (the Lord is a healer) works in and through all those involved in the healing process. I know that sometimes He even works without the use of my healthcare providers.

Whether through medical knowledge and skill or by divine intervention, my healing is for Your glory!

Amen

Rx

Meditate on faith

Read Hebrews 11:1

Pray with confidence and trust

A Prayer for Abnormal Growths

So Moses cried out to the LORD, "O God, please heal her!"

Numbers 12:13 (NIV)

Dear God I cry out as Moses did for Miriam's healing.

You created the parts of my body that make me uniquely female. My anatomy is diverse and specialized, cell by cell and layer upon layer.

Though You have designed and ordained the proper growth and function of each specific element of my body, there are many disruptions to this divine pattern that may result in masses, fibroids, cysts, tubal distortions, cervical lesions or other departures from Your original plan and purpose. These must be addressed and rectified.

Speak to my healthcare providers and give them the wisdom and skill needed to assist this healing process. I know that You are the master of all and that You work all things together for our good. You can transform abnormalities to comply with Your will and purpose by divine intervention or through my doctor's hands.

I bless and thank You for Your goodness and mercy with exceeding great joy!

To You be the glory and honor, forever!

Amen

R

Meditate on miraculous resolution

Read Daniel 4:2-3

Pray with expectation

Part III:
Prayers for Fertility

'Tis so sweet to trust in Jesus,

And to take Him at His word;

Just to rest upon His promise,

And to know, "Thus says the Lord!"[2]

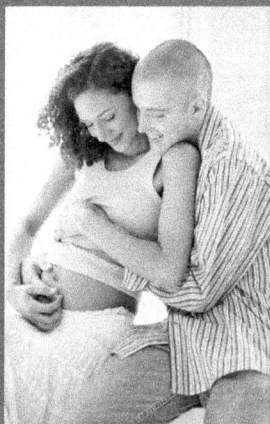
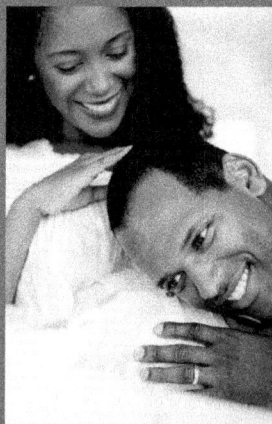
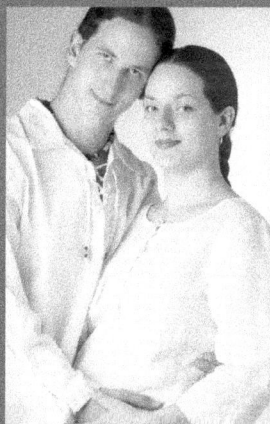

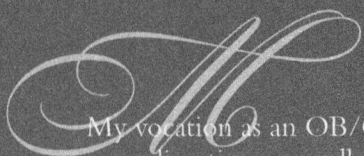

*M*y vocation as an OB/GYN has allowed me to walk with women during rewarding times as well as extremely difficult ones. As there are often no words to express the wondrous joy of giving birth, there are often no words to express the difficult task of telling an expectant couple that the pregnancy is not proceeding as hoped. It is just as difficult to deliver the dreadful report of yet another negative pregnancy test result to someone who has been attempting to get pregnant for years. Jesus said that He would not leave us comfortless (John 14:18). At these times when words seem entirely inadequate, prayer humbly offered can provide solace from the Great Comforter. Physicians are often called to minister to patients when medicine is not enough.

We can speak those things in prayer that are not manifested yet as though indeed they were (Romans 4:17). We can stand firm in the belief that the miraculous and supernatural can still happen. We can live in hope and declare and decree the future that God has for us.

The prayers that follow address a few of the more common circumstances that I have encountered in fertility challenges and difficult pregnancies over the years. They are the ones that often leave the healthcare provider, patient and family the most frustrated, distraught, confused and disappointed. It is important to remember that we can do all things through Christ who strengthens us (Philippians 4:13).

May God Almighty bless you and make you fruitful and increase your numbers . . .

Genesis 28:3 (NIV)

---

[2]*'Tis So Sweet to Trust in Jesus.* Lyrics by Louisa M. R. Stead (1882). Music by William J. Kirkpatrick (1882).

Part III:
Prayers for Fertility

A Prayer for Conception

God blessed them and said to them, "Be fruitful and increase in number; fill the earth and subdue it. . . ."

Genesis 1:28 (NIV)

O God, I stand in awesome wonder that You would grant me this tremendous honor and privilege to conceive and be the bearer of life as You give it. I worship You for who You are, the keeper of the soul, the restorer of the body, the renewer of the mind.

You have created the menstrual cycle to coordinate hormonal levels for the timely release of eggs and successful fertilization and preparation of the uterine lining for pregnancy. You have fashioned the uterus, tubes and ovaries to work together in glorious concert.

I stand in agreement with my healthcare providers that my body and reproductive capabilities will function as You have ordained for the purpose of conception. I stand against any process, conversation, thought or plan that is not aligned with Your divine purpose.

I know that there may be weapons that form, but they will not prosper. What You have ordained to be shall come to pass, and no demonic force shall prevail.

Grant wise counsel and sound medical judgment to all involved in my care. Let Your Holy Spirit permeate our homes, work environments and medical facilities. Your word states that You come to give life more abundantly (John 10:10)! I stand on that promise.

In You I live and move and have my being. In You new life will begin and move and have being (Acts 17:28).

Amen

Meditate on delighting in the Lord

Read Psalm 37:4

Pray with hope and adoration

A Prayer for Conception Healing

For I will restore health unto thee, and I will heal thee of thy wounds, saith the LORD . . .

Jeremiah 30:17 (KJV)

But he was wounded for our transgressions, he was bruised for our inequities: the chastisement of our peace was upon him; and with His stripes we are healed.

Isaiah 53:5 (KJV)

O Jehovah-Rophe (the Lord is a healer), I acknowledge You as the great healer and physician. I bless You, God, for You are all that I need—the great I AM (Exodus 3:14). You have provided the healing balm; indeed, You are the healing balm!

You have gifted doctors with the skills, knowledge and talent to provide healing, and You also heal miraculously by Your hand.

All healing is divine.

I come before You because there has been a disruption of what You have designed for the purpose of conception. The ovaries have not functioned appropriately or the fallopian tube has become dilated or distorted. This, God, is not of You, so I call these things back into divine order.

Where the uterine wall or lining has been disrupted so that it can no longer provide the nurturing environment for conception that You have decreed, I speak correction and healing to my body. If normal hormonal changes have become unbalanced, I speak divine balance and enhancement.

We can call those things that be not as though they were already in existence, and we operate on that principle (Romans 4:17). If there are any medical concerns with the future father, I ask that You reveal them to those who can assist with the diagnosis and treatment.

Instruct, enlighten and inspire all my healthcare providers to accurately treat as Your Holy Spirit directs. For those areas without any apparent explanation, I call on Jehovah-Mopheth (the God of Miracles).

Move, God, as only You can move and do what only You can do!

Amen

Ｒ𝚡

Meditate on the faithful One
who promised

Read Hebrews 11:11

Pray believing

A Prayer for Later Childbearing

The righteous will flourish like a palm tree, they will grow like a cedar of Lebanon; planted in the house of the LORD, they will flourish in the courts of our God. They will still bear fruit in old age, they will stay fresh and green, proclaiming, "The LORD is upright; he is my Rock, and there is no wickedness in him."

Psalm 92:12-15 (NIV)

God, Jehovah-Jireh (the Lord who provides), You hold everything in the palm of Your hand. I bless You God for who You are—great and majestic above all things.

You promise to restore the years that have been stolen from me (Joel 2:25). You promise to bless me abundantly above all I could ask, think or even imagine (Ephesians 3:20). You are the great Creator, and Your power is still immense and awesome. I place myself in Your faithful hands.

I will trust in You and delight myself in You, and You will give me the desires of my heart (Psalm 37:4). It is my desire to become pregnant. It is my desire to nurture life from conception to the first independent breath. It is also my desire to guide and protect this most precious infant through the growing years into adulthood.

I place this beloved baby in Your care from conception through eternity as You are the Alpha and Omega, and You know the end from the beginning. I will do all that I know to prepare my mind, body and spirit for this awesome task: to be a vessel for sacred service.

I ask for inspiration and enlightenment.

If there are challenges along the way, direct me to the appropriate medical consultants and spiritual counsel.

I align my mind and will to Your mind and will that Your purposes will be fulfilled. I cast down doubt, discouragement and lack during this process.

To God be the glory for this and all blessings in Jesus' name.

Amen

Rx

Meditate on great expectations

Read Ephesians 3:20

Pray knowing you shall receive

A Prayer for Early Pregnancy Loss

May the words of my mouth and the meditation of my heart be pleasing in your sight, O LORD, my Rock and my Redeemer.

Psalm 19:14 (NIV)

They remembered that God was their Rock, that God Most High was their Redeemer.

Psalm 78:35 (NIV)

O God, You are my strength and my redeemer!

You are my sword and my shield!

When I cannot see my way, You sustain and guide me. You are my comfort and my hope.

Though I may not understand what has happened or why, I know that You are in all things and will work them together for my good and Your glory.

As I go through this time of sorrow, confusion, pain and loss, I acknowledge my emotions, but, above them, I magnify You.

I stand on Your promises.

I touch and agree with my doctor and other healthcare providers that I will go through this process without significant bleeding, infection or other incident.

I decree that there will be no harm or injury to my reproductive anatomy.

I declare that my body, mind and spirit will be restored, renewed and invigorated for what is yet to come. I speak peace to myself and to those who are charged to care for my family and me during this time.

I ask that You give wise counsel and sound medical judgment to my healthcare team and that Your Holy Spirit abide in our homes, medical facilities and offices.

To God be the glory for what He has done and will do!

Amen

Rx

Meditate on being sustained by God's promises

Read Psalm 55:22

Pray and hold to God's promises

A Prayer for Recurrent Pregnancy Loss

O LORD, our Lord, How excellent is Your name in all the earth, Who have set Your glory above the heavens! Out of the mouth of babes and nursing infants You have ordained strength, Because of Your enemies, That You may silence the enemy and the avenger.

Psalm 8:1-2 (NKJV)

O God, my God, my heart is heavy and my spirit is hurting, but I will yet praise You in this experience. Though I have many questions, I do not have the answers as to why this happened again, but I will continue to trust You.

It is my desire to be pregnant and to give birth to a healthy child.

I know that this is Your will for me because You have fearfully and wonderfully made my body for this purpose. You have designed my ovaries and tubes to accommodate conception. You have designed the process necessary for hormonal balance to support pregnancy. You have designed my uterus to be a sanctuary for the development and maturation of the pregnancy, and You intricately orchestrated the process that leads to labor and delivery.

As I go through this time of sorrow, confusion and loss, I acknowledge my emotions, but, above them, I magnify You. I stand on Your promises and the word You have given to me.

I touch and agree with my doctor and other healthcare providers to silence the enemy of doubt, anger, unbelief and strife in our homes, medical facilities and offices.

I align my mind to the mind of Christ and cast down the works of the evildoer.

Supply wise counsel and sound medical judgment, and let Your Holy Spirit abide with me as I seek to do Your will and give You all the glory!

O LORD, our Lord, How excellent is Your name in all the earth!

Psalm 8:9 (NKJV)

Amen

℞

Meditate on God's mercy and truth

Read Psalm 57:1

Pray for understanding and discernment

Part IV:
Prayers for Pregnancy Health

Behold, I am the LORD, the God of all flesh: is there any thing too hard for me?

Jeremiah 32:27 (KJV)

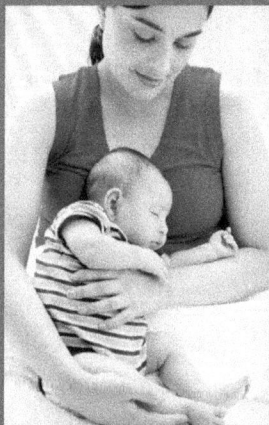

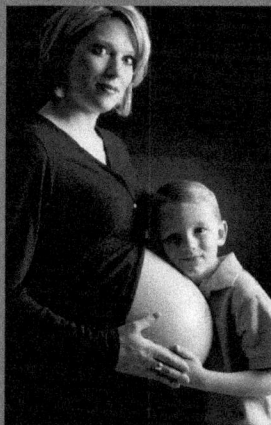

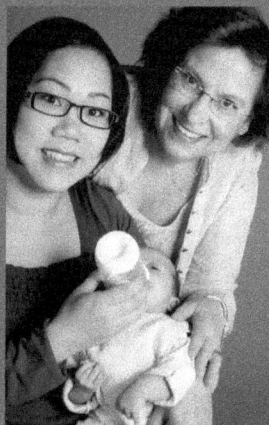

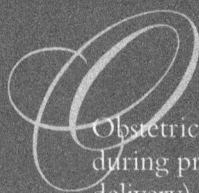

Obstetrics (the branch of medicine that deals with the care of women during pregnancy, childbirth and the recuperative period following delivery) is both rewarding and challenging. Most expectant mothers have normal and healthy pregnancies and deliveries. However, there are times when pregnant women come to me with preexisting medical disorders such as diabetes, hypertension or obesity. There are also several problems that can occur that are unique to pregnancy such as preeclampsia, an incompetent cervix or preterm labor. In these instances, obstetricians will frequently partner with maternal fetal medicine specialists as well as other highly trained medical and surgical consultants. A healthy outcome of these pregnancies is facilitated through a team effort.

Though medicine utilizes protocols and scientific evidence, it is also very much a healing art. Healing is divine in nature. Many dedicated doctors recognize the need for a power greater than themselves. "Is any one of you sick? He should call the elders of the church to pray over him and anoint him with oil in the name of the Lord. And the prayer offered in faith will make the sick person well" (James 5:14-15, NIV).

I do not believe that it is "either-or" when it comes to seeking medical attention and having faith in God to heal and sustain. Rather, I ascribe to faith in God Almighty for divine intervention and in His Spirit who works in and through the medical profession. When medical and surgical techniques are placed in God's hands, they become divine tools that bring about health.

But he was pierced for our transgressions, he was crushed for our iniquities; the punishment that brought us peace was upon him, and by his wounds we are healed.

Isaiah 53:5 (NIV)

Part IV:
Prayers for Pregnancy Health

A Prayer for Diabetes in Pregnancy

For I will give you words and wisdom that none of your adversaries will be able to resist or contradict.

Luke 21:15 (NIV)

O Lord, by Your divine design many hormonal changes are necessary for normal growth and development during pregnancy. There can sometimes be an increase in certain placental hormones that interfere with the body's normal use of insulin, which leads to abnormal blood sugar levels.

I ask that You reveal any alterations that may result in pregnancy-related diabetes or that may worsen preexisting diabetes. Speak to all of my doctors and other healthcare providers, and move by Your divine hand to maintain the normal intrauterine environment necessary for my baby's normal development.

Dear God, whether Your hands heal directly or through the combination of diet, activity and medication, I will look to Your words for wisdom and instruction. Give my family guidance, and make my home environment one that reflects Your divine will and purpose for this pregnancy.

To God be the glory!

Amen

℞

Meditate on being redeemed

Read Isaiah 43:1

Pray for balance
and perseverance

A Prayer for High Blood Pressure in Pregnancy

. . . "Daughter, your faith has healed you. Go in peace."

Luke 8:48 (NIV)

Jehovah-Rophe (the Lord is a healer), I acknowledge that there is nothing too hard for You!

Whether existing before the pregnancy or manifesting during the pregnancy, there are problems with my blood pressure that must be addressed.

My doctors and other healthcare providers understand that various physiological changes can occur during pregnancy that affect the cardiovascular system and the kidneys. There are many other organs that can also be affected by blood pressure elevations.

God, You can normalize these biochemical reactions and vascular changes through my doctors with medications and changes in my diet and my exercise regimen, as well as divinely by Your hand.

Protect my baby and my intrauterine environment as a blessed sanctuary. Protect me so that I suffer no hurt or injury that circumvents my divine purpose as a parent. I am called to lead this precious one through infancy to adulthood.

Give my doctors and other healthcare providers a heightened sense of kairos (divine time).

I speak healing and peace.

In Jesus' Name.

Amen

R_x

Meditate on the words
"I am healed"

Read Isaiah 53:5

Pray for stability and normalcy

A Prayer for Cervical Disorders

You will be secure, because there is hope; you will look about you and take your rest in safety.

Job 11:18 (NIV)

O God, You have wonderfully and intricately designed my body to function for reproduction.

There has perhaps been some traumatic injury, hormonal disruption or congenital change that led to the premature opening of the cervix. Guide my doctors and other healthcare providers as decisions are made about whether to use surgery or other conservative measures for management.

My security and hope are in You.

If necessary for me to be treated, dispatch Your ministering angels about my healthcare facilities.

Let Your Holy Spirit go before and with me.

Keep me ever mindful that I will lie down and sleep in peace, for You alone, O Lord, make me dwell in safety.

In Jesus' name.

Amen

℞

Meditate on God's help in times of trouble

Read Psalm 30:2

Pray for strength and integrity

A Prayer for Preterm Labor

But when the time had fully come, God sent his Son . . .

Galatians 4:4 (NIV)

My Lord, You are the God of exquisite and specific timing.

Your word is full of references to set times, appointed times and the fullness of time. Truly our times are in Your hands as is the perfect timing for my baby's birth.

I take authority over possible causes for early labor including infection or anatomical abnormalities of the womb. No one cause has been isolated in all instances of preterm labor, but You are Jehovah Elohim (Supreme God).

I speak peace to the waves of contractions to calm the uterus as Jesus spoke "peace, be still" to the waves of the storm.

Guide my doctors and other healthcare providers should it become necessary for me to have frequent examinations, cervical assessment, uterine monitoring or for them to limit my activity. It may become necessary to use medications to stop the uterine contractions or steroids to help accelerate my baby's ability to breathe when born.

In all of this, my hope and trust are ultimately placed in You and Your kairos (divine time).

May Your Peace and Holy Spirit rule.

Amen

℞

Meditate on peace and rest

Read Exodus 14:14

Pray for health and divine functioning

A Prayer for Intrauterine Growth Restriction (IUGR)

And in him you too are being built together to become a dwelling in which God lives by his Spirit.

Ephesians 2:22 (NIV)

My God, You designed the placenta with its many layers, proteins and transport systems to provide nutrition throughout pregnancy and to clear unwanted materials.

Many processes work in concert with my body, placenta and developing fetus to ensure that this transfer of nutrients and oxygen takes place unimpeded.

I stand against any disruption or compromise that is leading to my baby's abnormal growth. I declare that the injury or cause is arrested and reversed now to allow for the proper, divinely ordained flow.

El Shaddai (God Almighty), I call on Your abundant source, my wellspring, to provide all that my baby needs to grow, develop and flourish. I specifically speak to my kidney system for the production of normal fluid levels and to the oxygenation of the brain and nervous tissue that coordinate proper organ function.

Give inspiration and revelation to my doctors and other healthcare providers as they monitor everything closely to determine the appointed time for safe delivery.

For Your glory and honor.

Amen

R_x

Meditate on thriving and flourishing

Read Psalm 92:12

Pray for increase

A Prayer for Preterm Loss of Fluid

He calms the storm, So that its waves are still.

Psalm 107:29 (NKJV)

. . .And you shall be called the Repairer of the Breach, The Restorer of Streets to Dwell In.

Isaiah 58:12 (NKJV)

Adonai (Lord, Master), You calm the seas, and You can also take charge of this situation.

The actual cause for this early leaking of fluid from around my baby may be attributed to many factors. Perhaps it is due to a decrease in the blood supply of the membranes or because of some disruption of their inner layers.

Whatever the cause, I call everything into divine order from this time forward. I speak to the blood supply as well as the collagen-rich matrix between the membrane layers that protect my baby from injury.

Prevent any compromise to my baby by prolonging the pregnancy as long as necessary, allowing Your creative process to complete its work.

Divinely protect my baby and me from infection, and give special insight to the doctors and other healthcare providers who are watching over me and my precious harvest of love.

To God be the glory.

Amen

℞

Meditate on shelter

Read Psalm 27:5

Pray for restoration

Part V:
Prayers for the Expectant Father, Pregnancy and Delivery

. . . and the LORD enabled her to conceive, and she gave birth . . .

Ruth 4:13 (NIV)

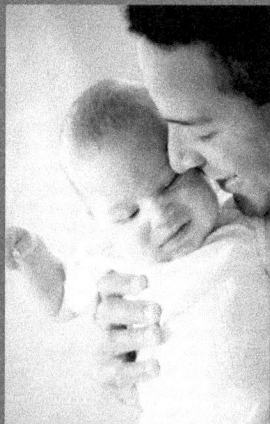
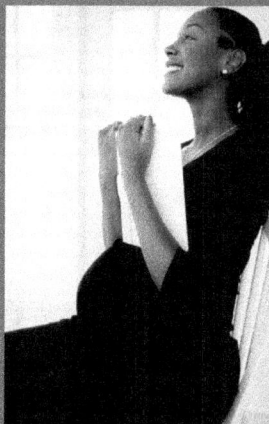
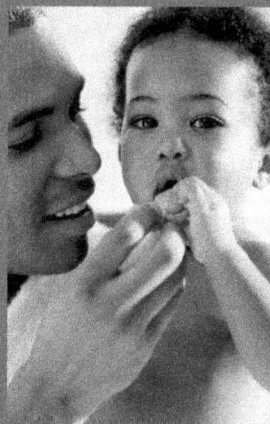

The wonders of pregnancy and birth never cease to amaze me because of the intricate details involved from conception to labor to birth. There is no doubt in my mind that God's divine hand is controlling the whole process, from the initiation of that special chemistry between two people who become one in love to holding the result of that love for the first time.

I bless God for the opportunity that He has afforded me to be present when babies take their last internal breath in their mother's womb to their first independent one in this world, truly an Alpha and Omega moment— a miracle! I give honor and praise to God, for I know that I can only do what I do because of what He has already done.

He has made everything beautiful in its time. He has also set eternity in the hearts of men; yet they cannot fathom what God has done from beginning to end. I know that there is nothing better for men than to be happy and do good while they live.

Ecclesiastes 3:11-12 (NIV)

Part V:
Prayers for the Expectant Father, Pregnancy and Delivery

A Prayer for the Expectant Father

Blessed is the man who does not walk in the counsel of the wicked or stand in the way of sinners or sit in the seat of mockers. But his delight is in the law of the LORD, and on his law he meditates day and night. He is like a tree planted by streams of water, which yields its fruit in season and whose leaf does not wither. Whatever he does prospers.

Psalm 1:1-3 (NIV)

O God, I bless and praise You for ordaining the parentage of this child.

Just as Jesus acknowledged You, our Father in heaven, so I recognize and honor my baby's father. He is an awesome man of God who has been called into our lives to lead, protect, comfort and provide.

As he submits to Your will, so I will submit to him.

Through You, let him be a steadying rock and a shoulder to lean on throughout this pregnancy.

I will continue to need him in the days, weeks and years to come to guide our child, Your fruit, to his or her divine purpose and destiny.

May You continue to bless and protect my baby's father. Strengthen and anoint him for the greater work yet to come.

To God be the glory forever!

Amen

R

Meditate on the man of God

Read Genesis 17:4-6

Pray earnestly as needed

Month One

For you created my inmost being; you knit me together in my mother's womb.

Psalm 139:13 (NIV)

And It Begins!

Thank You God for what You have already done!

I marvel at Your divine hand in creation.

From the moment that the unique microscopic elements combined to bring about this life, You supplied everything that was needed to form every organ and system. Even eye and hair colors have already been determined. Every detail of the body is truly fearfully and wonderfully made.

I am thankful for this journey to motherhood and for the process that started even before pregnancy to prepare my uterus to be a home for my baby's development.

Though I may not look or even feel pregnant, much is going on to ensure a healthy outcome: blood vessels are forming, the nervous system's intricate connections are being made on a molecular level and hormonal coordination of the entire process is under way.

I rely on Your divine protection as You orchestrate this delicate process.

Holy Spirit speak to my doctor and other healthcare providers, and give them divine revelation and guidance. As I am instructed, I will be very careful to follow all guidelines for nutrition, activity, supplements and medications.

I speak to the ovaries and placental layers needed for normal hormone productions and for the implantation of the embryo into its new dwelling place.

I seek to rest in the shadow of the Almighty, and I commit my course to You.

You will bring successful completion of this pregnancy!

To God be the Glory!

Amen

R_x

Meditate on a new beginning

Read Genesis 2:7

Pray for abundance

Month Two

The Spirit of God has made me; the breath of the Almighty gives me life.

Job 33:4 (NIV)

Dear God, incredible transformations are taking place now. Your divine plan has ordained that the umbilical cord is thick and strong as it fulfills its function of carrying vital nutrients and oxygen between my baby and me.

Numerous cells and layers are beginning to develop into different organs and systems. The nerve cells are growing that will coordinate their functioning, and the eyes are beginning to form that will see so many wonders in the weeks and years to come. During this month, tiny buds for the hands and feet will form, and, most amazingly, the tiny heart will beat rapidly.

My heart is already full of love for this life You have given.

All the glory and honor is Yours, for it is by Your mercy and Your grace.

Holy Spirit, You have entrusted my care to knowledgeable and compassionate doctors. Rest, rule and abide in their medical offices so that peace will be waiting there for my baby and me.

Speak to my doctors continuously. Bless and keep them and their homes and families.

We know that the enemy may by lurking, seeking whom he may devour, but Your power reigns supreme to protect that which You have created.

You are a faithful God, and my baby and I are in Your care.

May all that You have ordained during this critical developmental period come to pass without harm or injury.

Make my body and home a blessed sanctuary for Your creative process.

In Jesus' Name.

Amen

R_x

Meditate on being purposefully formed by God

Read Psalm 139:13

Pray for completeness

Month Three

Ears that hear and eyes that see–The LORD has made them both.

Proverbs 20:12 (NIV)

My Lord and my God, my mind cannot sometimes comprehend all that has happened in these first weeks.

Your grace and splendor are overwhelming, as is the delicacy of Your divine design.

The building components for bones and muscles are starting to surround and support tiny, fragile organs, and the elements that will form ears are developing their form and function. Therefore, even now I speak life and love to this precious being for its hearing.

As You are molding and strengthening my baby's internal frame and balance, also strengthen my relationships with my loved ones. As my baby's father and I were a unit in the creation of this life, keep us together and draw us closer to each other and to You.

What God has joined together, let no one put asunder (Matthew 19:6).

I speak peace and protection.

I know that angels have already been dispatched to aid my baby and me.

Have my doctors and other healthcare providers keep careful watch over Your delicate works. Bless their eyes to see what needs to be seen and their ears to hear what needs to be heard.

Amen

R̽

Meditate on wonderful work

Read Psalm 139:14

Pray for no lack or abundance

Month Four

"I am the vine; you are the branches. If a man remains in me and I in him, he will bear much fruit; apart from me you can do nothing."

John 15:5 (NIV)

O my Lord, what is happening to me now is becoming so real. I can see the evidence of my baby's growth within, and I want to continue to grow spiritually.

I need You more now than ever as I face certain medical decisions. I know that You are the source of life and wisdom.

Speak to my baby's father and me as we consult with all of my healthcare providers. Give them the wisdom and insight to provide necessary information for our consideration. Bless them and keep them. Let peace rule!

If I were to peek inside now, I would be able to see if this is a boy or girl. Miraculous changes are happening that will continue to mold my baby into a wonderful individual.

Unique fingerprints are forming, and every hair is numbered by You.

I remain awed and humbled by Your majesty and benevolence.

Continue to be my wellspring—my abundant source.

In Jesus' name.

Amen

Rx

Meditate on wisdom

Read 1 Kings 4:29

Pray for understanding

Month Five

'For in him we live and move and have our being . . .

Acts 17:28 (NIV)

Glorious God, how wonderful it is to live and move in You as I can now feel my baby moving inside of me.

You are great and wonderful, and I never want to take for granted all that You have done.

What a wonder it is to know that as my baby moves, connections and nerve development for physical and mental processes that are important now and after birth are being established.

Small muscles are getting stronger, and my baby's body is beginning to fill out and grow. So it is as I grow and mature in You.

All that has happened before to develop the depth of my relationship with You has been for me to fulfill this special purpose for my life.

Continue to inspire me to do all that is needed to ensure the healthy growth and development of my baby.

You designed my uterus to be a sanctuary for this purpose alone. It serves no other.

I declare that Your will be done.

Let Your Holy Spirit permeate the offices and medical facilities that I will visit, and give revelation to my doctor and other healthcare providers when necessary.

I recognize and respect the education and talent that You have blessed them with, but there is so much that remains unknown. Indeed, there are many mysteries of life.

Continue to protect and keep this small life from all hurt, harm or danger, seen and unseen, and protect me as I travel about.

In Jesus' name.

Amen

℞

Meditate on protection

Read Psalm 5:11

Pray for confidence in God

Month Six

. . . because he himself gives all men life and breath and everything else.

Acts 17:25 (NIV)

O Lord, I speak life to this precious one through Your Holy Spirit and power.

My baby is now just a miniature version of what he or she will look like at birth.

By Your declaration, everything just continues to get stronger, more developed and specialized and weight gain is rapid. I can tell that my baby's hearing is more acute because external sounds like my voice lead to a responsive movement.

My baby's movements can be felt from outside when hands are placed on my abdomen.

What a miracle! What an awesome experience!

My baby's lungs and chest muscles begin to practice breathing movements in preparation for the first external breath, but that time is not now.

My womb needs to remain stable and quiet, for labor is yet to come.

For now I speak, "Peace, be still."

There are tests that may need to be done at this point, and I expect a good report.

I reverence You, God, for Your mercy and Your grace.

More visits are needed now, for that expected end is getting closer.

Keep my doctor and other healthcare providers ever vigilant and watchful over this great harvest. Weapons may form, but none will prosper for the Lord stands ready as

Jehovah-Nissi (the Lord is my banner),

Jehovah-M'Kaddesh (the Lord who sanctifies),

El Shaddai (God Almighty),

By Your power I live.

Amen

R

Meditate on peace

Read Philippians 4:7

Pray for blessed assurance

Month Seven

Blessed are the pure in heart, for they will see God.

Matthew 5:8 (NIV)

El Roi (God of seeing), You are the God who opens our eyes and who assigns vision and purpose.

During this time, my baby's eyelids begin to open and close, and the nerve connections that allow for sight are functioning.

Even at this time, You can give vision.

I speak purpose and meaning over this most precious life that his or her spiritual vision will be sharp and discerning.

O God, as You hold and keep this life, whisper purpose even now into my baby's innermost parts. Make Your vision for my baby's life clear to me and to all those who will influence him or her.

My baby's father and I acknowledge that we must remain focused on You so that we can rightly fulfill our purpose as parents.

Let us never forget that You are the abundant source, the wellspring, from which we draw. You are the true vine. Keep our hearts pure that we may continue to see You in every aspect of our lives.

As a deer pants for the streams of water, so our souls pant for You, O God! We need Your protection and Your guidance (Psalm 42:1).

Your holy presence is the essential thing.

Keep us in Your sight.

Amen

Rx

Meditate on vision and purpose

Read Habakkuk 2:2

Pray for destiny to be fulfilled

Month Eight

But they that wait upon the LORD shall renew their strength; they shall mount up with wings as eagles; they shall run, and not be weary; and they shall walk, and not faint.

Isaiah 40:31 (KJV)

O God, how great You are, for You are He who indwells, sanctifies, searches the heart and gives life.

You designed my body to provide my baby with the appropriate nutrition and protection from disease during this important time.

Everything in my baby's body is preparing for entry into the world. The developmental process for the lungs, brain and nervous system continues and is near completion.

I am making preparations, and my doctors and other healthcare providers are following everything closely.

This is a time of patiently waiting with hopeful anticipation.

Lord, I keep my mind on You.

Calm any fear or anxiety, and settle any frayed emotions.

Though much has already been done, there are still a few tasks yet to be completed.

I speak Your word and know that it will not return to You void or unfulfilled. It will accomplish that for which it was sent (Isaiah 55:11).

Thy will be done!

Amen

R℞

Meditate on maturation

Read James 1:4

Pray knowing God will provide

A Prayer as Time Draws Near

. . . "Blessed are you among women, and blessed is the child you will bear!"

Luke 1:42 (NIV)

As toys, clothes, furniture and showers of blessings are being planned, God, I offer up this prayer that You are in all that is done.

I pray that Your Holy Spirit will permeate every thought, deed and gift and that You continue to protect, nurture and hold this precious life in safekeeping. Strengthen my body that it may remain a blessed sanctuary for Your creative work to be completed.

My excitement and anticipation are building as I await the entrance of this miraculous gift.

Go before me in this process and prepare the way. Bless all of the healthcare facilities, doctors, nurses and other healthcare personnel that You have entrusted with the care of my baby and me.

Continue to speak to my baby's father, my family and me, and reveal Your will to us.

Give us wise spiritual and medical counsel as we stand together with my healthcare providers. Together we are a community of faith.

We are committed to providing all that we can for this child as we are led by Your Holy Spirit. Bless and keep us in Your will.

To God be the Glory!

Amen

R

Meditate on patient expectation

Read Psalm 62:5

Pray for the capacity to endure

Month Nine

Now the LORD was gracious to Sarah as he had said, and the LORD did for Sarah what he had promised.
Genesis 21:1 (NIV)

So in the course of time Hannah conceived and gave birth to a son . . .
1 Samuel 1:20 (NIV)

Then God remembered Rachel; he listened to her and opened her womb.
Genesis 30:22 (NIV)

In Due Time!

Dear Lord, the wonder of giving birth has been taking place since the beginning of time. My trust is in You and in those in whose care I have been placed.

There are no accidents, and there is nothing unknown to You. You are Alpha and Omega, the beginning and the end (Revelation 1:8).

You are Jehovah-Rohi (the Lord is a shepherd) who will guide and protect me through this marvelous experience.

I call on You, for You are faithful, willing and able.

You are

Adonai (Lord, Master),

Jehovah-Shammah (the Lord is there),

Jehovah-Shalom (the Lord is peace),

El Elyon (Most High),

El Olam (Everlasting God),

El Berith (God of the Covenant).

All is ready! My baby waits to make an entrance and be celebrated at birth.

May all proceed according to Your divine design and timing, without peril or incident.

Angels have assumed their posts around the delivery facility. Your Holy Spirit is resting on all of the doctors, nurses and other attendants.

I bring peace and will meet peace when I arrive.

I celebrate the cycle of pregnancy that is ending and the circle of life that is beginning.

To God be the glory.

Forever and ever.

Amen

Meditate on new life

Read Job 33:4

Pray with hopeful anticipation

~ Closing ~

My life experiences have brought me to this point where prayer is an essential element for me to survive. I have gained much and lost some during my existence, and I have concluded that if I lose my relationship with God, nothing else truly matters.

I hope that this book has helped to provide a framework to encourage women and their families to strengthen their own personal relationships with God, to study His Word and to pray very specifically for any medical issues that concern them.

I pray that the perceived divide between living a life of intellectual excellence and living a life filled with faith and spiritual authority will disappear. It is my hope that this work helps to facilitate that process and that it serves as a starting point for prayers regarding other medical concerns.

We are in a very real spiritual battle and are told that "the weapons we fight with are not the weapons of the world. On the contrary, they have divine power to demolish strongholds" (2 Corinthians 10:4, NIV). Further, Ephesians 6:12 (NIV) confirms that "our struggle is not against flesh and blood, but against the rulers, against the authorities, against the powers of this dark world and against the spiritual forces of evil in the heavenly realms."

Though we may not be biblical scholars or seminarians, we are all encouraged to fill ourselves with God's word so that when the fiery darts are sent in our direction, they can be deflected, and we can walk in our divine purposes. Jesus instructs us not to dwell in vain repetitions when seeking revelation and guidance from God through prayer (Matthew 6:7); rather, through a sincere and open heart, He instructs us to place our concerns before Him and patiently wait in His presence for divine insight and direction in all that is needed.

I close with this prayer from my heart:

May your pursuit of God and a bountiful prayer life intensify so that you will prosper and be in health even as your soul prospers (3 John 1:2). May the anointing of the Holy Spirit be released in your life through prayer for your health and well-being. May your heart's desire be fulfilled abundantly and the peace of God surround you completely. May the redeeming and powerful blood of Jesus protect you and strengthen you to do all that God has purposed for your life, and may the fruit of your body be blessed and empowered for eternity.

Now to him who is able to do immeasurably more than all we ask or imagine, according to his power that is at work within us, to him be glory in the church and in Christ Jesus throughout all generations, for ever and ever! Amen.

Ephesians 3:20-21 (NIV)

Appendix A:
Devotional Scriptures for
Part I: Prayers for Women at the Well

Yeshua (Messiah)–John 1:41, 4:25-26, 4:42

Kinsman Redeemer–Job 19:25, Isaiah 44:6

Sanctifies–1 Thessalonians 5:23, 1 Peter 1:2

Forgiveness–Luke 7:44-48, Psalm 103:1-5

Speak life–Psalm 118:17

Fountain of life–Psalm 36:9

God with her–Psalm 46:4-5

Give many days–Deuteronomy 11:20-22

Appendix B:
Devotional Scriptures for
Part II: Prayers for Gynecologic Health

Healing balm–Psalm 147:3; Luke 6:18-20

Abundance of the heart–Luke 6:45

Imaginations–2 Corinthians 10:5

No respecter of persons–Acts 10:34

Jehovah-Rophe (the Lord is a healer)–Exodus 15:26, Jeremiah 30:17

Gifts of healing–1 Corinthians 12:9, 12:27-31

God is creator–Isaiah 44:24, 64:8; Colossians 1:15-17

Giver of blessings–Psalm 84:11

Wisdom–Proverbs 16:22, 18:4

Healing in His wings–Malachi 4:2

Healed–Isaiah 53:5; Psalm 107:20

Appendix C:
Devotional Scriptures for
Part III: Prayers for Fertility

Fearfully and wonderfully made–Psalm 139:14

Abundant life–John 10:10

Breath of life–Genesis 2:7

Maker of all things–Ecclesiastes 11:5

God's promises–2 Corinthians 7:1; Romans 15:7-9

Renewed strength–Isaiah 40:31

Bind and loose–Matthew 16:19

Jehovah-Jireh (The Lord who provides)–Genesis 22:4

Restorer–Joel 2:25

Delight in the Lord–Psalm 37:4

Waiting for God–Isaiah 8:17

Abundant blessings–Ephesians 3:20, 21

Meet your needs–Philippians 4:19

Equip you for His will–Hebrews 13:20-21

Sarah–Genesis 21:1-2

Rebekah–Genesis 25:21

Rachel–Genesis 30:22-23

Hannah–1 Samuel 1:18-20

Shunammite woman–2 Kings 4:12-17

Elizabeth–Luke 1:24-25

Appendix D:
Devotional Scriptures for
Part IV: Prayers for Pregnancy Health

Alpha and Omega–Revelations 1:8

Shadow of the Almighty–Psalm 91:1-2

Appointed time–Psalm 102:13

Sanctuary–Exodus 15:17-18

Love overflows–1 Thessalonians 3:12-13

Strong relationships–Matthew 19:4-6

Hairs numbered–Matthew 10:27-31; Luke 12:6-8

Maturity–1 Peter 2:1-3

Jehovah-Nissi (The Lord is my banner)–Exodus 17:15

El Shaddai (God Almighty)–Genesis 17:1-2; 28:3

Peace, be still–Mark 4:39

Showers of blessings–Ezekiel 34:26

In the womb–Psalm 71:6

True vine–John 15:5

Soul yearns for God–Psalm 42:1

Blessings for offspring–Deuteronomy 7:13-5; Psalm 127:3-5; Isaiah 44:2-5

Faithful–2 Thessalonians 3:3; Psalm 119:90

Childbirth–John 16:21

Jehovah-Rohi (The Lord is a shepherd)–Psalm 23 1-6

Adonai (Lord, Master)–Genesis 15:2

Jehovah-Shammah (The Lord is there)–Ezekiel 48:35

Jehovah-Shalom (The Lord is peace)–Leviticus 7:11–21

El Elyon (Most High)–Genesis 14:18-20; Psalm 78:35

El Olam (Everlasting God)–Genesis 21:33; Psalm 90:1-3; Isaiah 26:4

El Berith (God of the Covenant)–Genesis 12:2-3; Exodus 19:5

Appendix E:
Devotional Scriptures for
Part V: Prayers for the Expectant Father,
Pregnancy and Delivery

Plans for your life—Jeremiah 29:11-13

Faith that heals—Luke 8:48

God's word—Isaiah 55:11

Flourish—Psalm 92:12

Stilled the storm—Psalm 107:29

Completed time—Galatians 4:4

Only wise God—Jude 1:24-25

All things are possible—Matthew 19:26

Heals all diseases—Psalm 103:3

Confidence in God—1 John 5:14-15

Encouraged to pray—Philippians 4:6

Notes

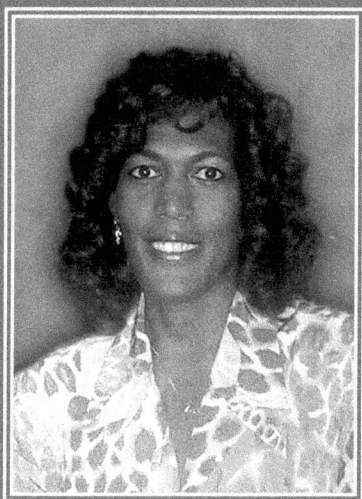

∽ About the Author ∽

Mironda D. Williams, M.D., is a board certified obstetrician and gynecologist and a graduate of Cornell University and Morehouse School of Medicine. While completing her medical residency at the Medical College of Georgia, Dr. Williams was appointed the first Black female chief resident of obstetrics and gynecology. A native of Atlanta, Dr. Williams is a partner in a successful obstetrics and gynecology practice in the Atlanta metropolitan area and the founder of MD WELLSPRING, an organization dedicated to the vision for medicine and miracles. The cornerstone of Dr. Williams' practice is state-of-the-art medical intervention, spiritual revelation and passionate prayer. Dr. Williams is a dedicated church member and community volunteer.

You may contact Dr. Williams at info@mdwellspring.com.

Books may be ordered by e-mailing orders@mdwellspring.com.

*This book offers
God-inspired prayers for women
struggling with gynecologic health
problems that result in disease
and the inability to become pregnant
and give birth. It also contains
prayers for health during each month
of pregnancy. The goal of this book
is to renew women's faith in God's
power to heal and work miracles.*

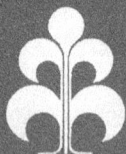

MD WELLSPRING

www.ingramcontent.com/pod-product-compliance
Lightning Source LLC
Chambersburg PA
CBHW071338290326
41933CB00039B/1665